Bands

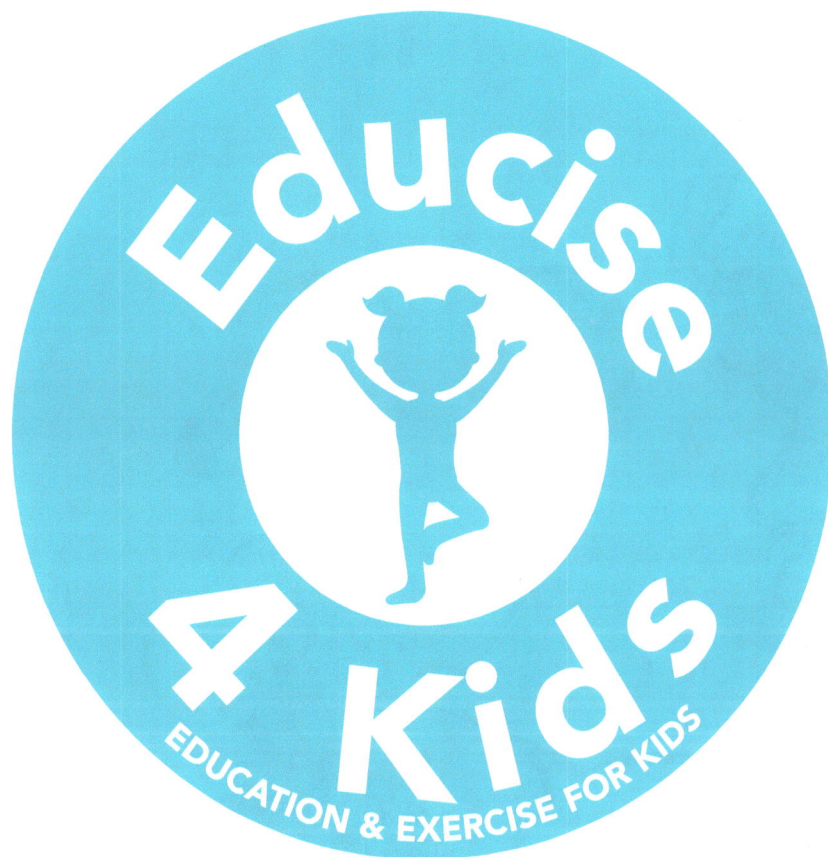

Created By
Priscilla Fauvette

Illustrated By
Bernard Fauvette

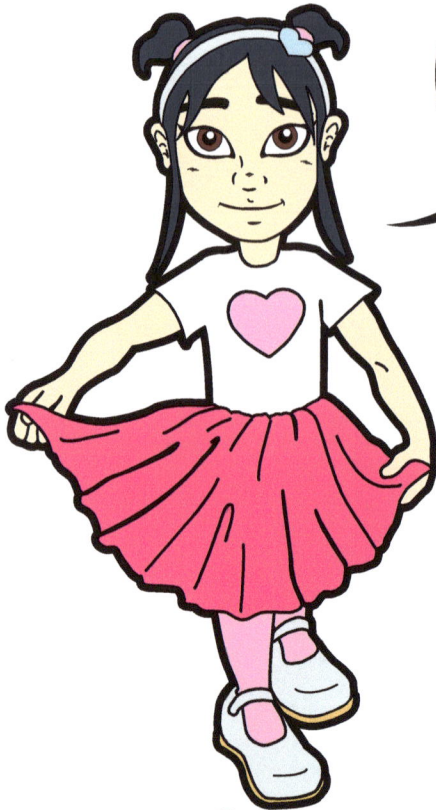

MAKE TIME FOR REST & RELAXATION

LIN

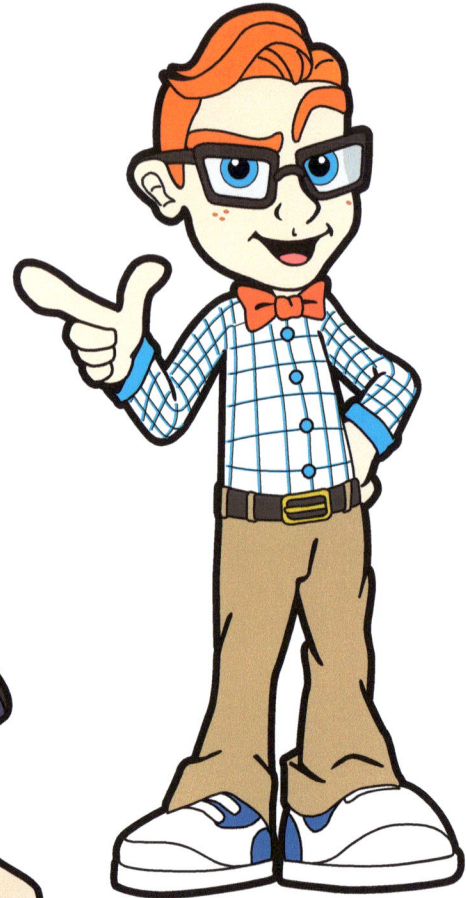

CADEN

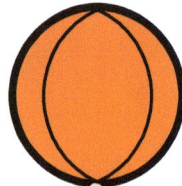

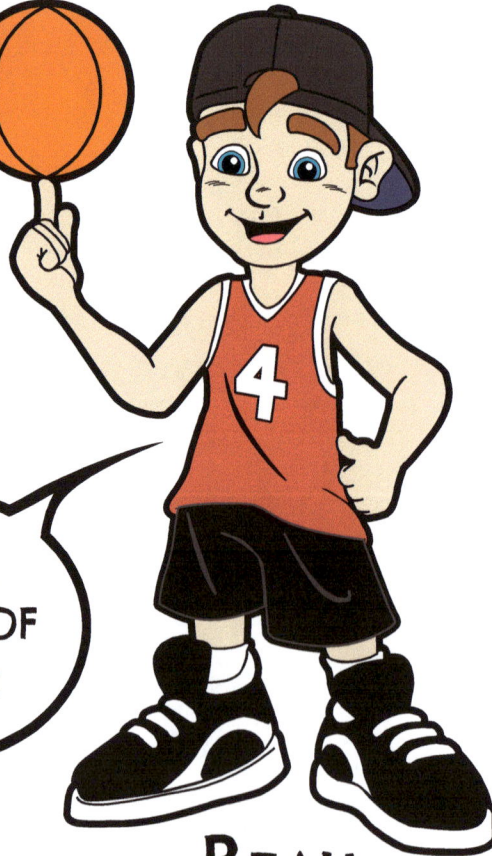

DRINK PLENTY OF WATER

BEAU

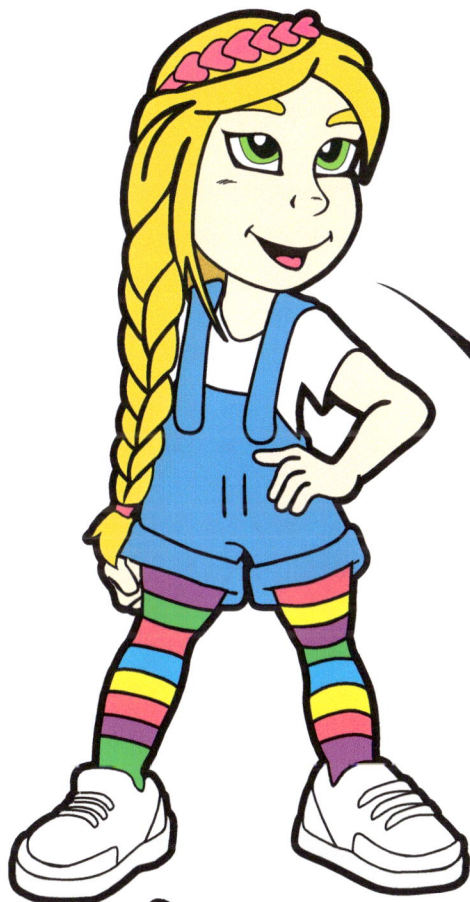

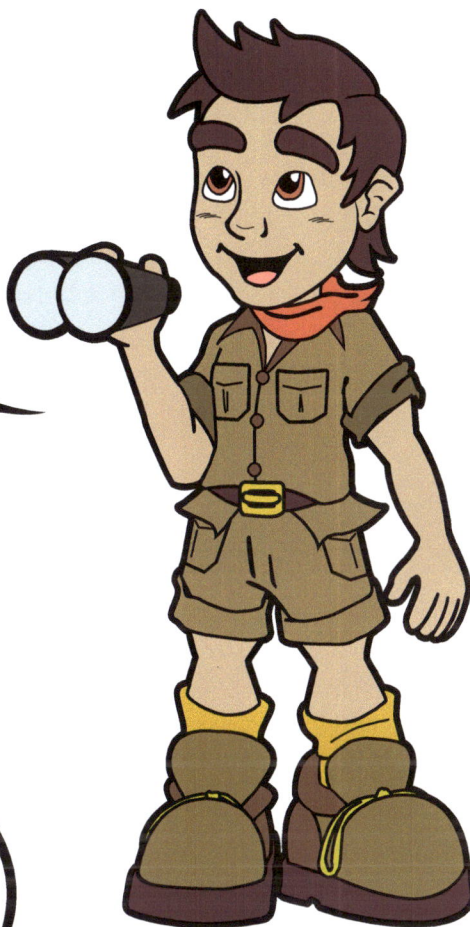

Anatomy

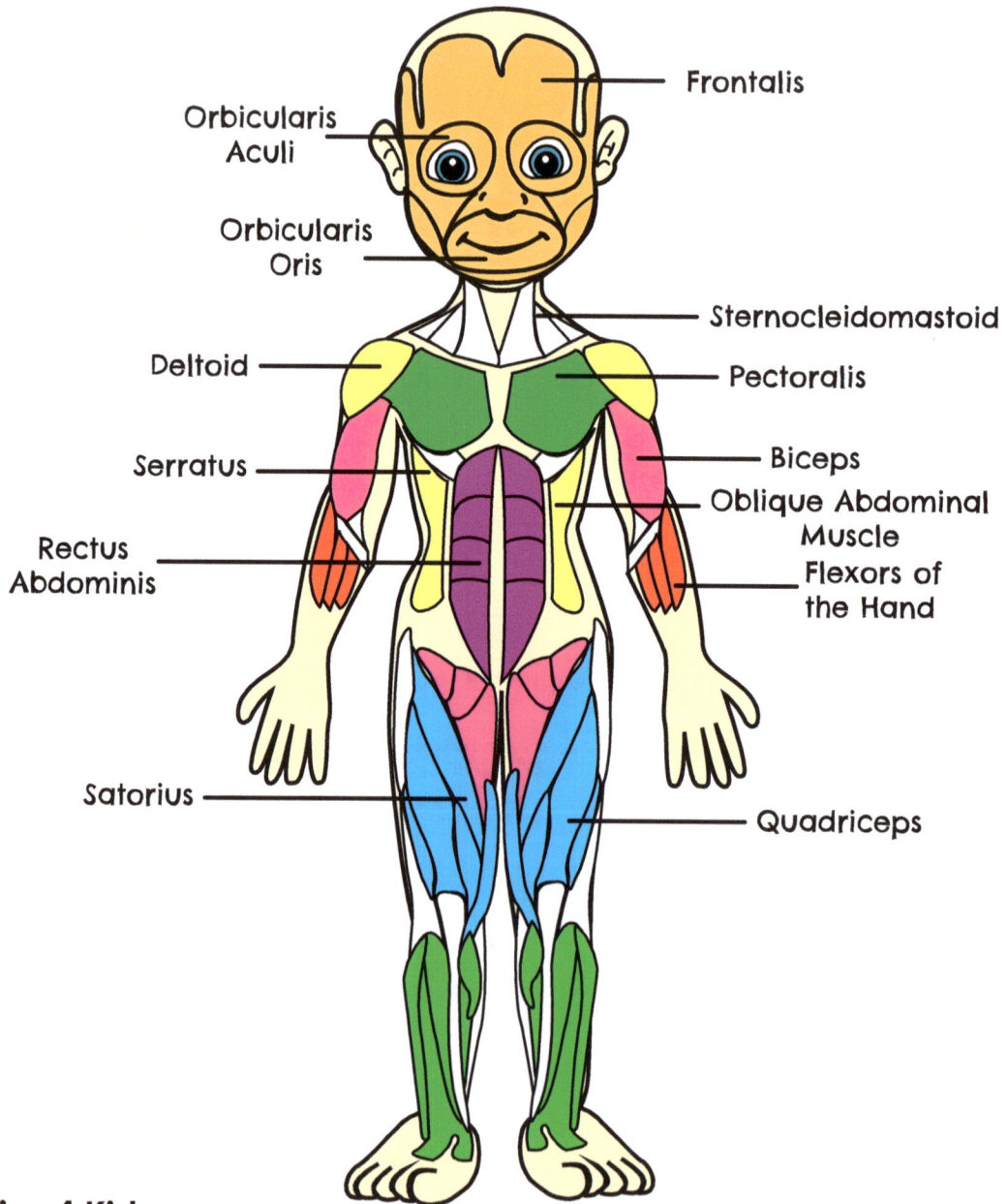

Frontalis

Orbicularis
Aculi

Orbicularis
Oris

Sternocleidomastoid

Deltoid

Pectoralis

Serratus

Biceps

Oblique Abdominal
Muscle

Rectus
Abdominis

Flexors of
the Hand

Satorius

Quadriceps

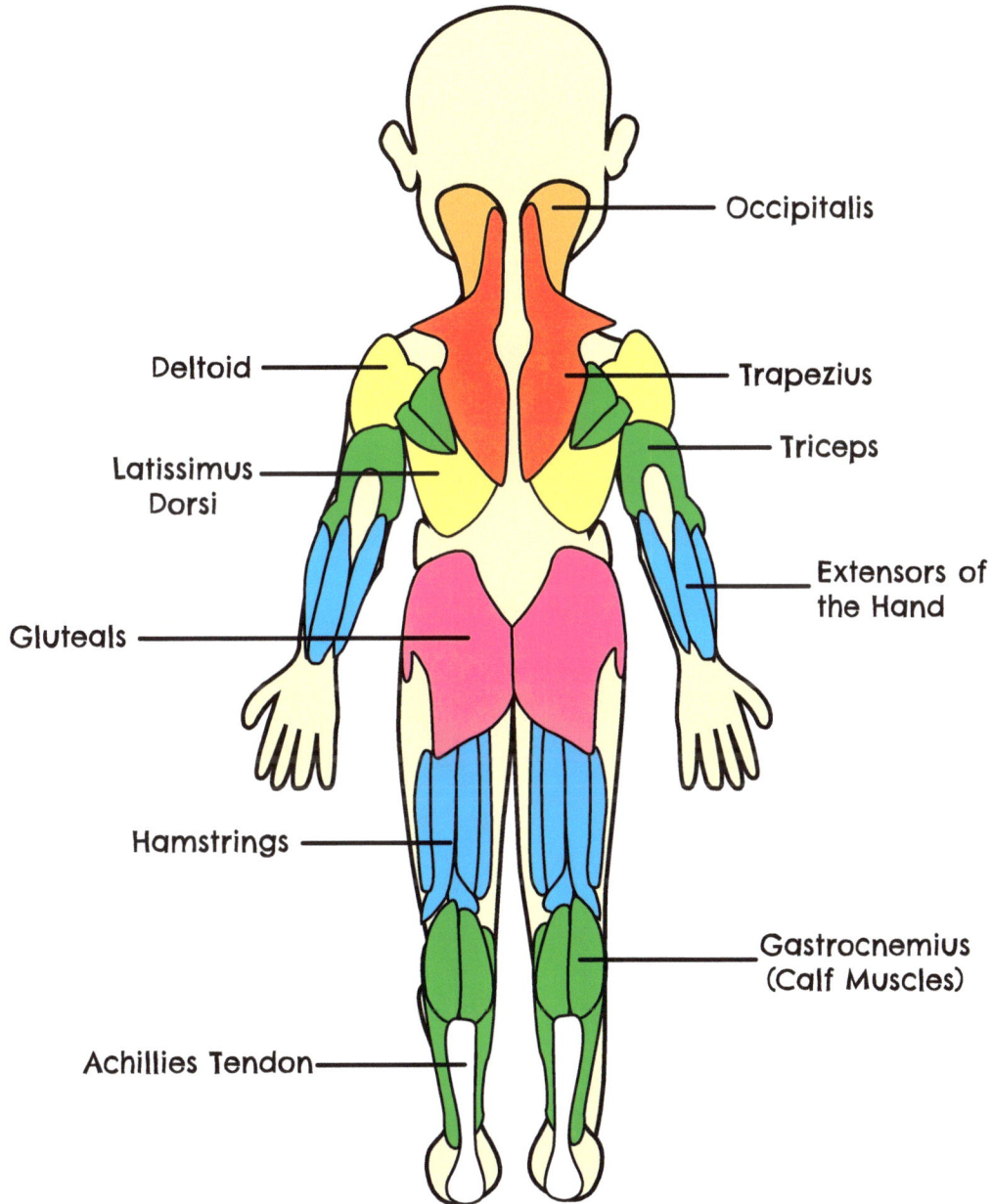

Anatomy

Occipitalis

Deltoid

Trapezius

Triceps

Latissimus Dorsi

Gluteals

Extensors of the Hand

Hamstrings

Gastrocnemius (Calf Muscles)

Achillies Tendon

Upright Rows

Stand up tall

Place your band under your feet

Hold the band in your hands

Cross the bands over

Keep your arms in front of your body

Slowly bring your elbows up high

above your shoulders

Lower them back down to the first position

Can you do this 5 times?

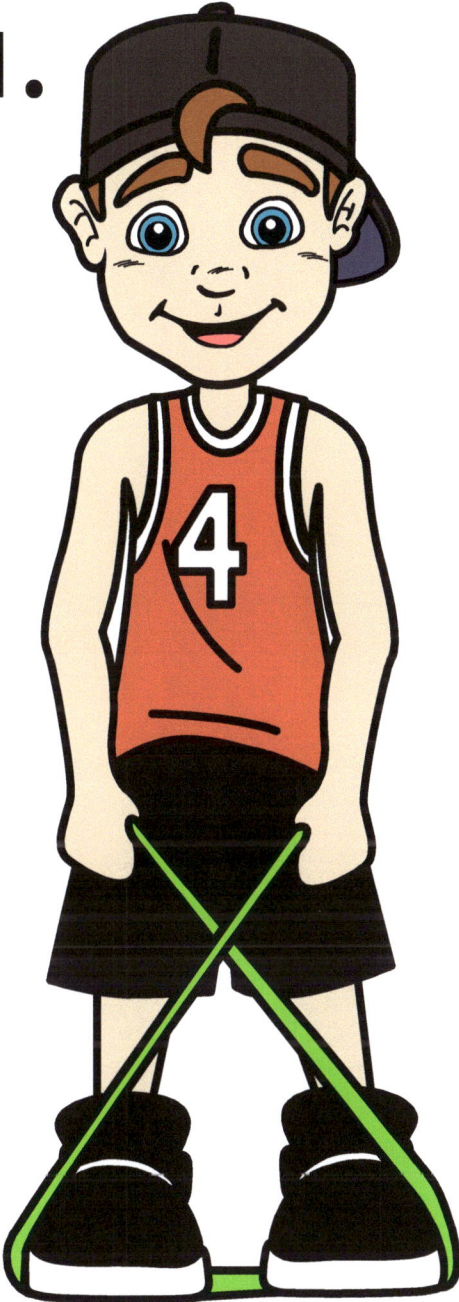

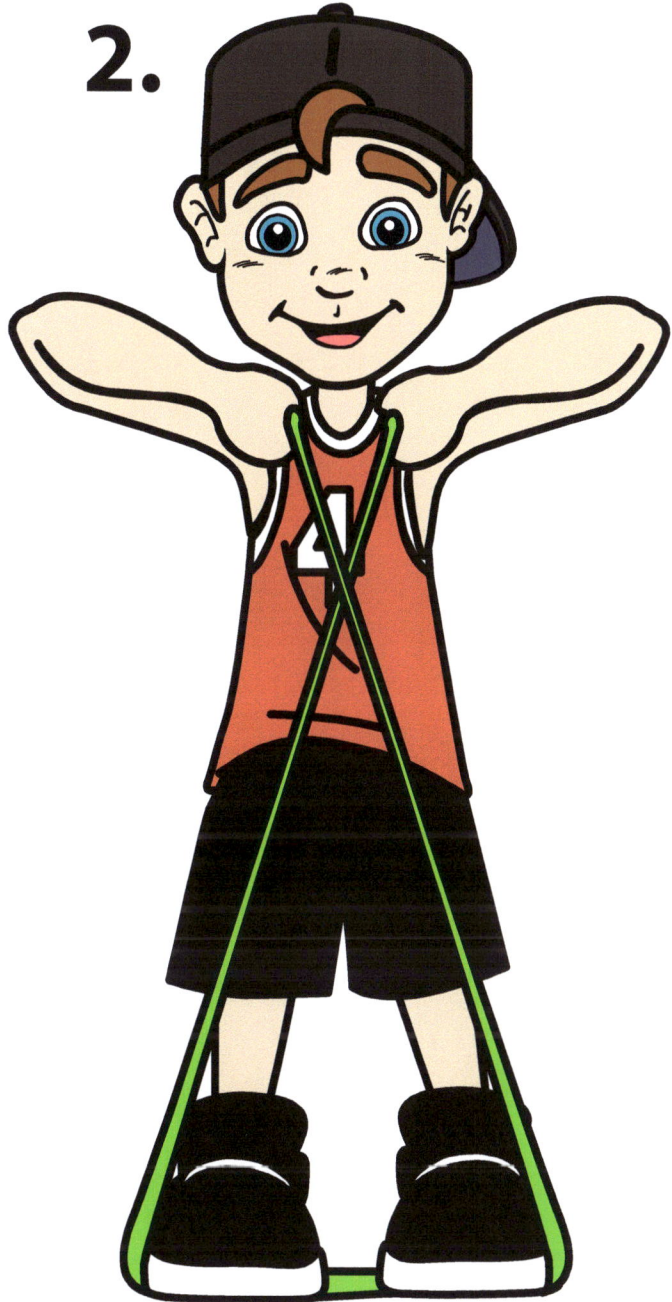

1.

2.

Tricep Kick Backs

Stand up tall

Place the band under your feet

Hold the band in your hands

Keep your arms in front of your body

Bend your upper body over slightly

Keep your elbows close to your body

Slowly bring your hands away from your body

Now bring your hands back down

Can you do this 5 times?

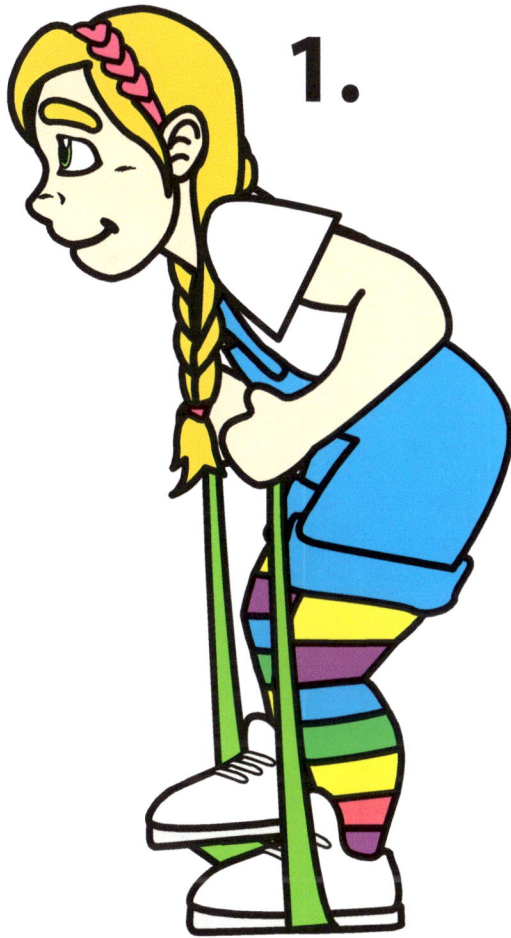

1.

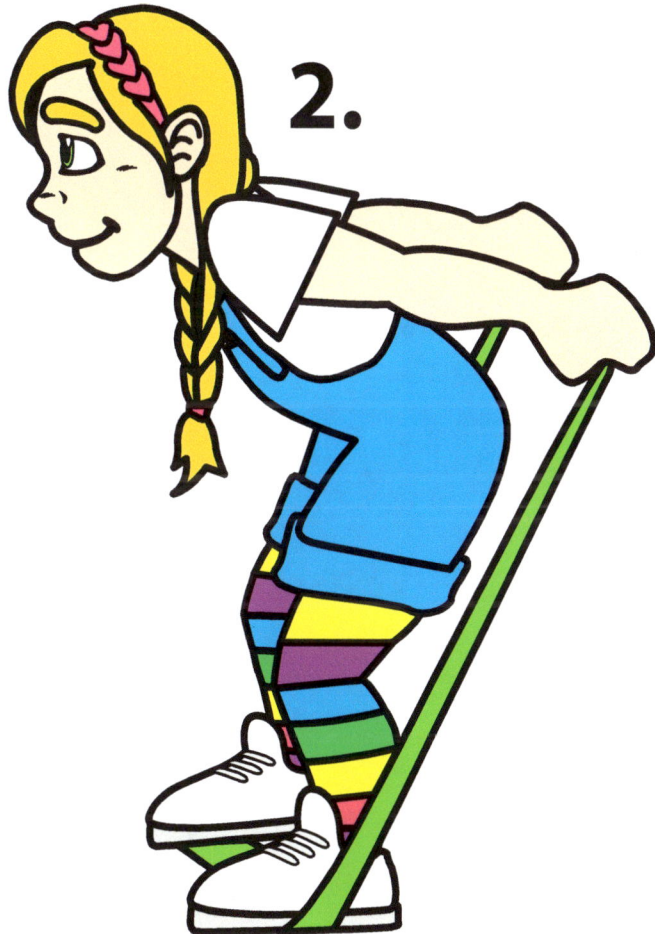

2.

Frontal Raises

Stand up tall

Place the band under your feet

Hold the band in your hands

Keep your arms in front of your body

Slowly bring your arms upwards

Lower your arms back to your side

Can you do this 5 times?

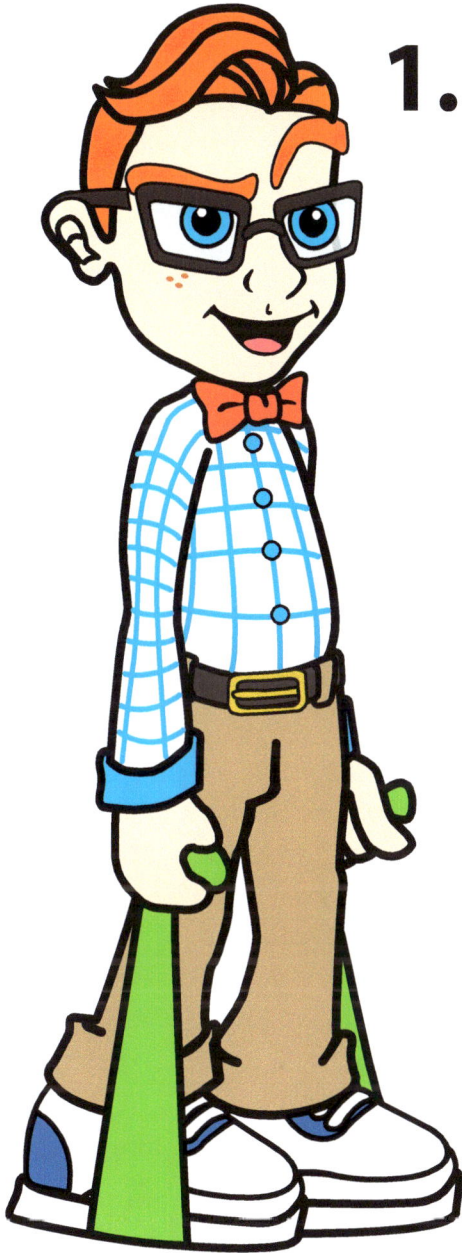

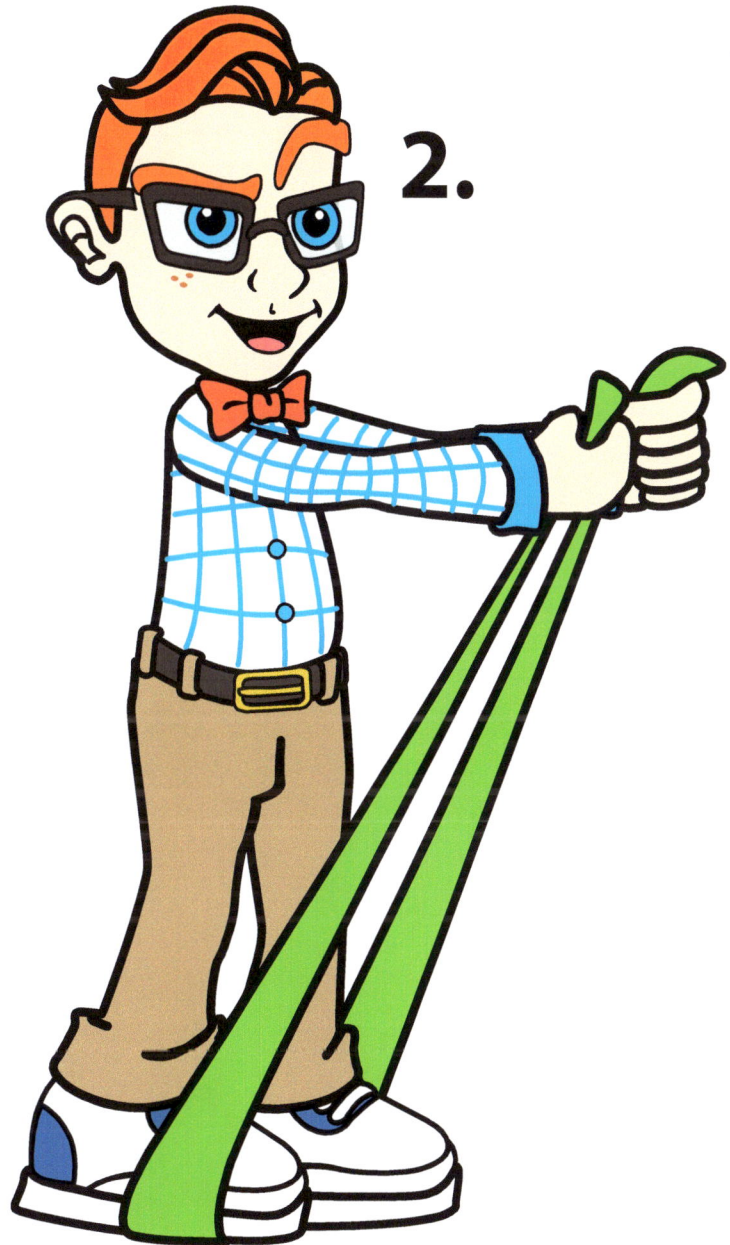

1.

2.

Lateral Raises

Stand up tall

Place the band under your feet

Hold the band in your hands

Keep your arms in front of your body

Slowly bring your arms out sideways

Keep your arms straight and
your elbows slightly bent

Lower your arms back to the start

Can you do this 5 times?

1.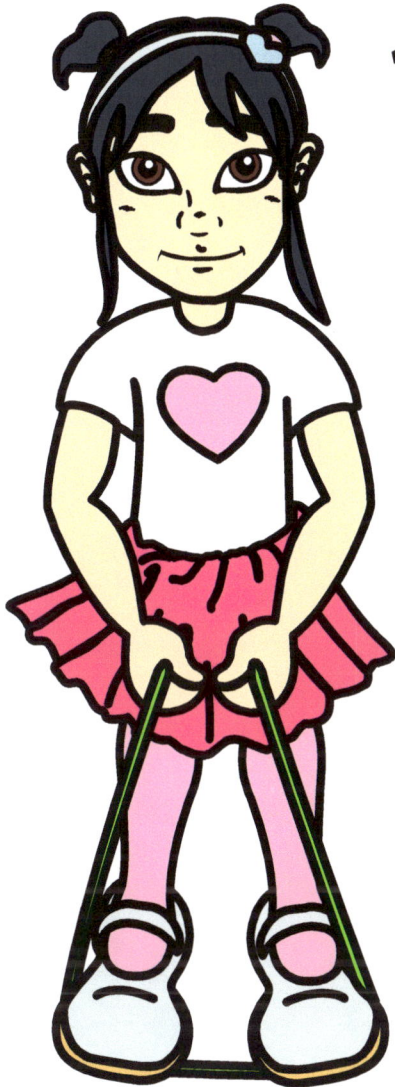

2.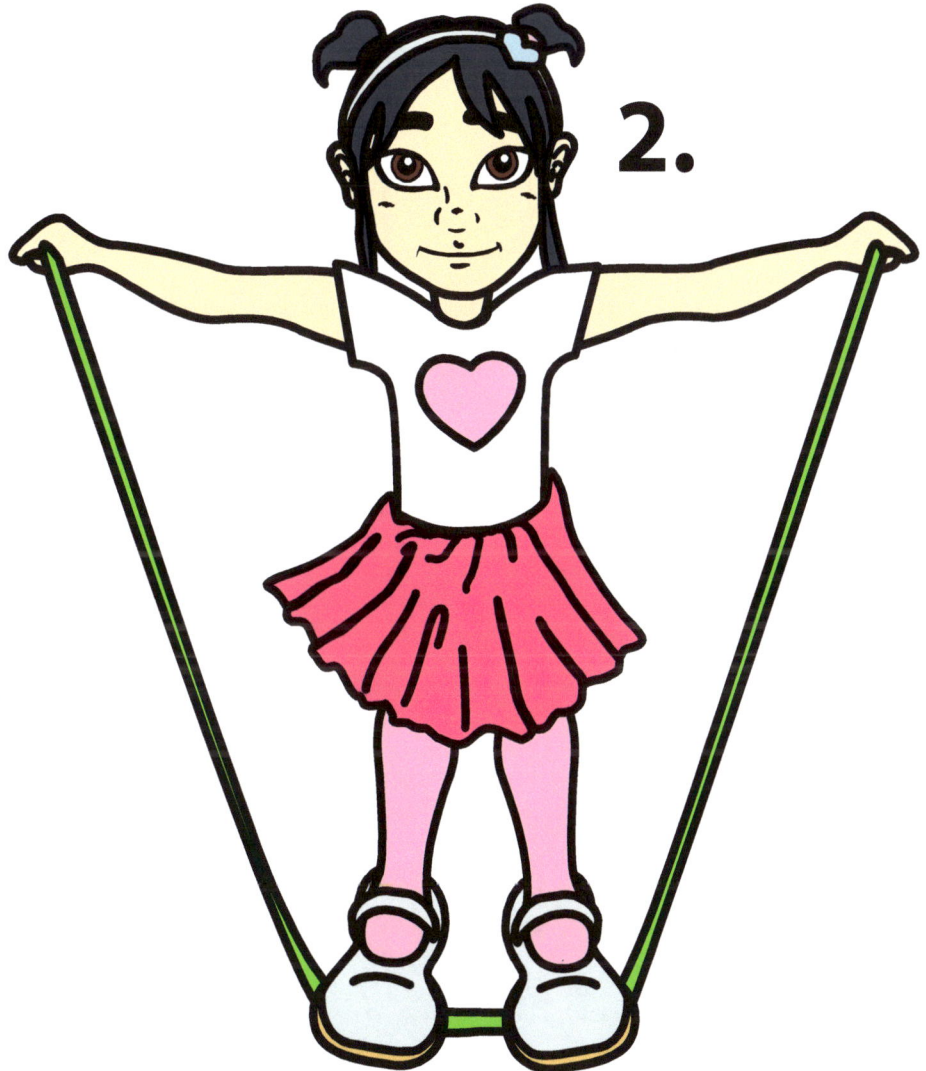

Lunges

Stand up tall

Take one step forward

Place the band under your front foot

Hold the band in your hands

Slowly lower your back leg

Raise your arms with the band at the same time

Keep your back straight

Now push yourself back up again

Can you do this 5 times?

1.

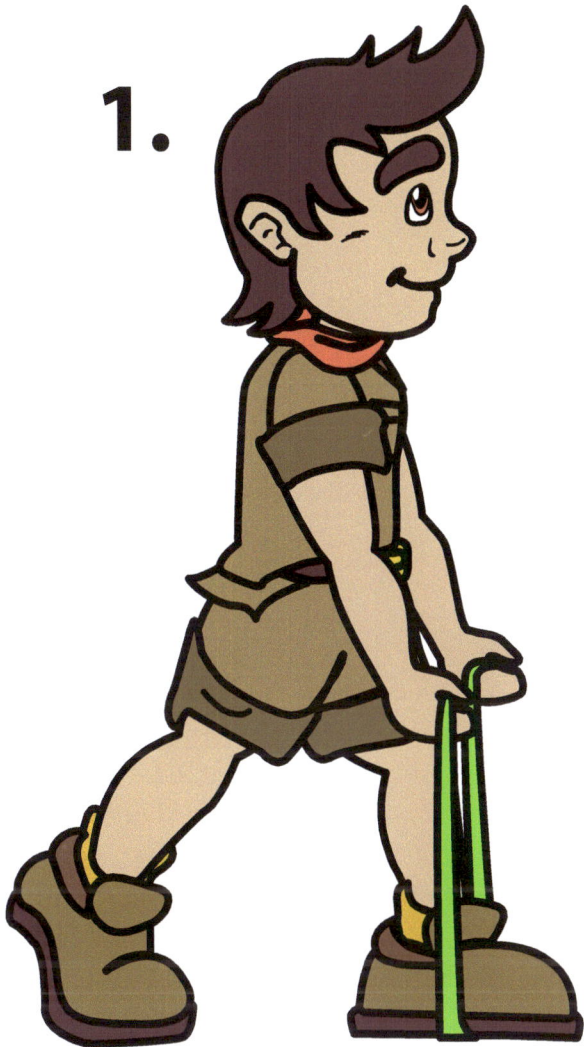

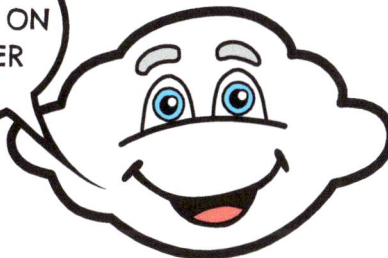

2.

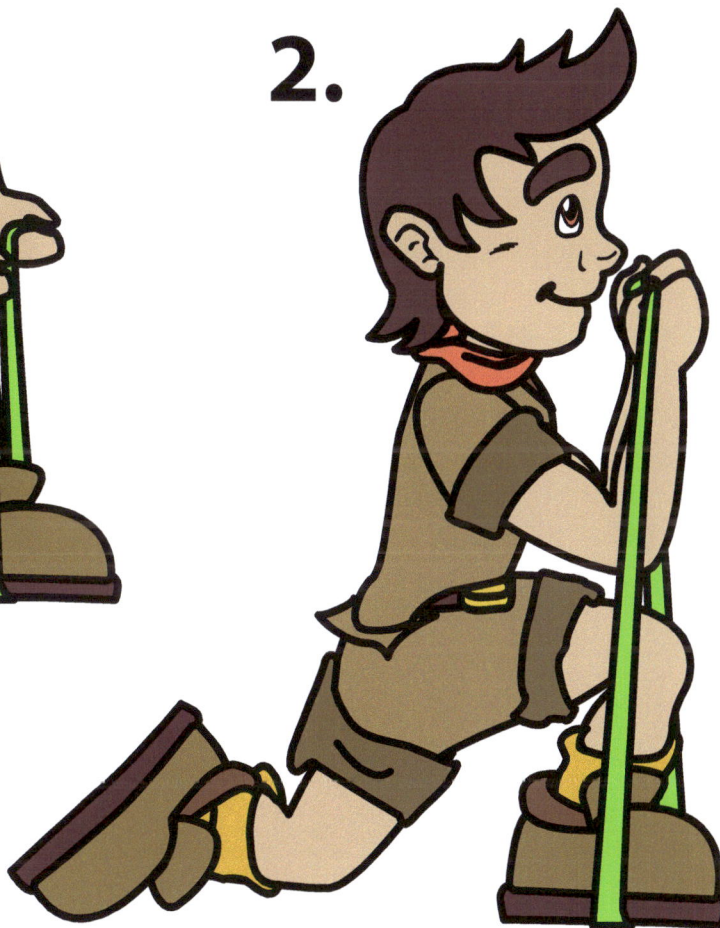

Push Ups

Lay flat on the floor

Place the band around your back

Hold the band with your hands

Place your hands beside your body

Push your whole body up

Keeps your arms and back straight

Slowly lower your body back down

Can you do this 5 times?

1.

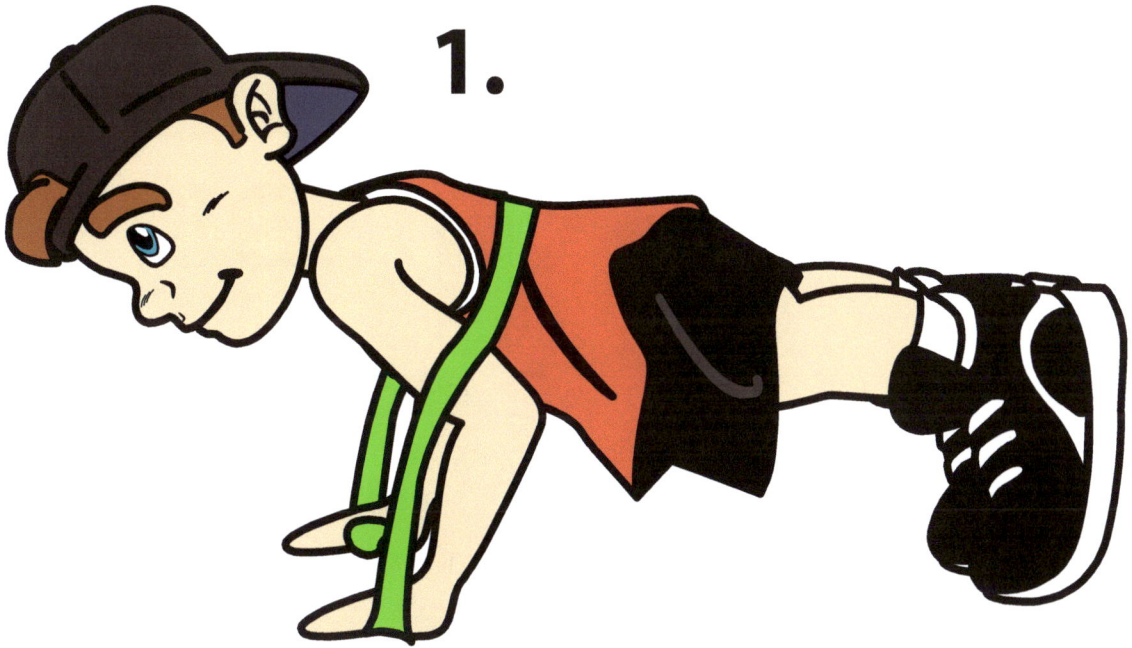

2.

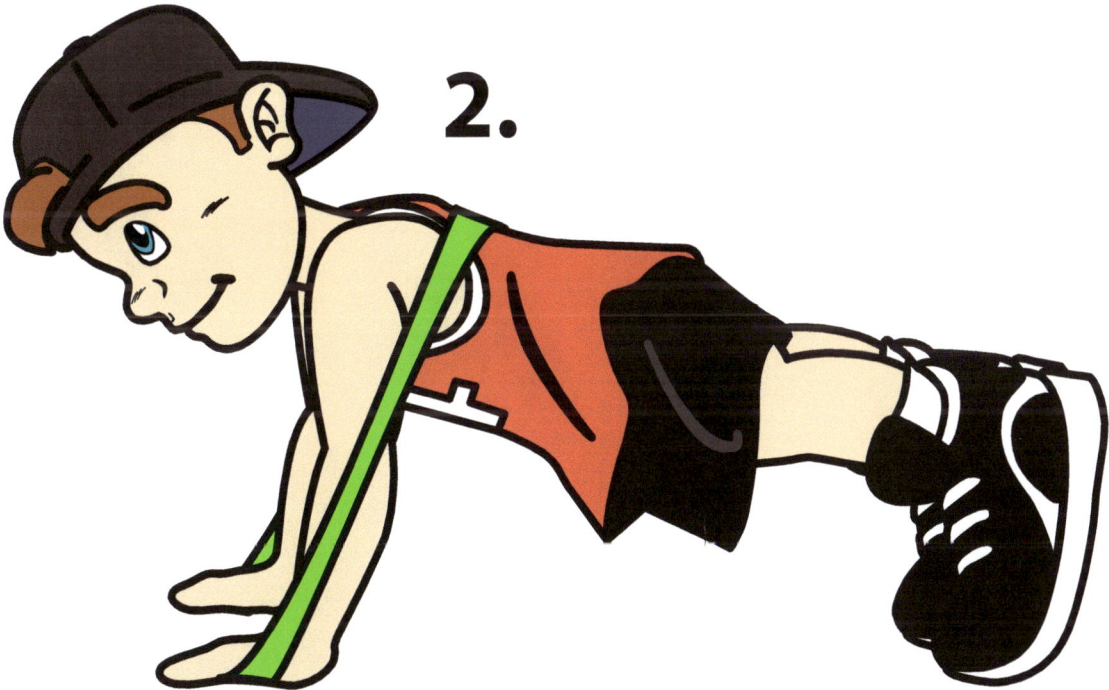

Calf Raises

Sit on the floor

Bend one leg and keep the other straight

Place the band over the top part of your foot

Hold the band with your hands

Slowly point your toe forward

Bring your toe slowly back

Can you do this 5 times?

1.

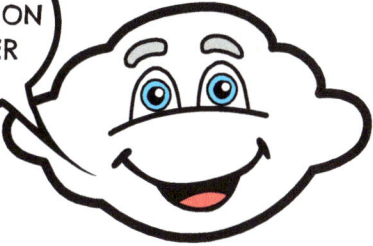

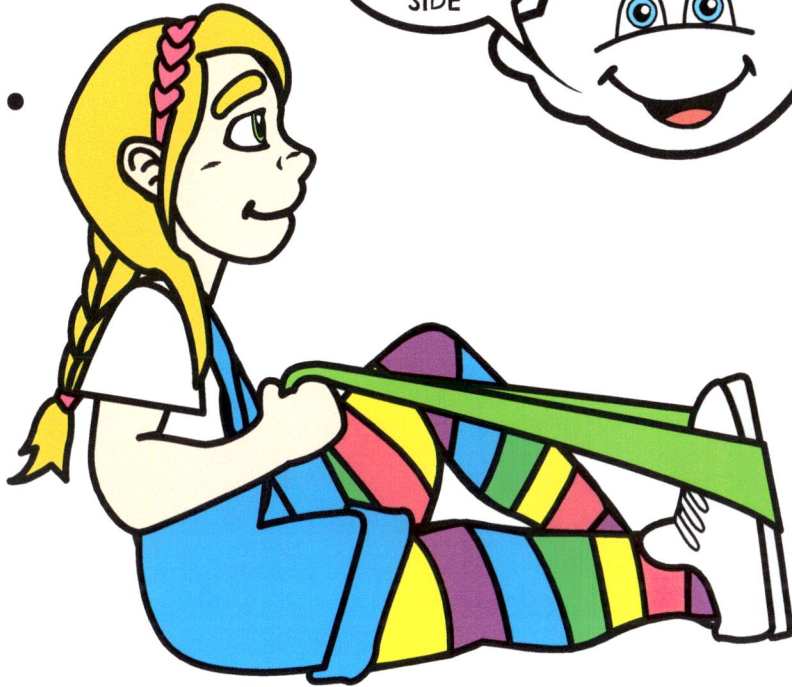

2.

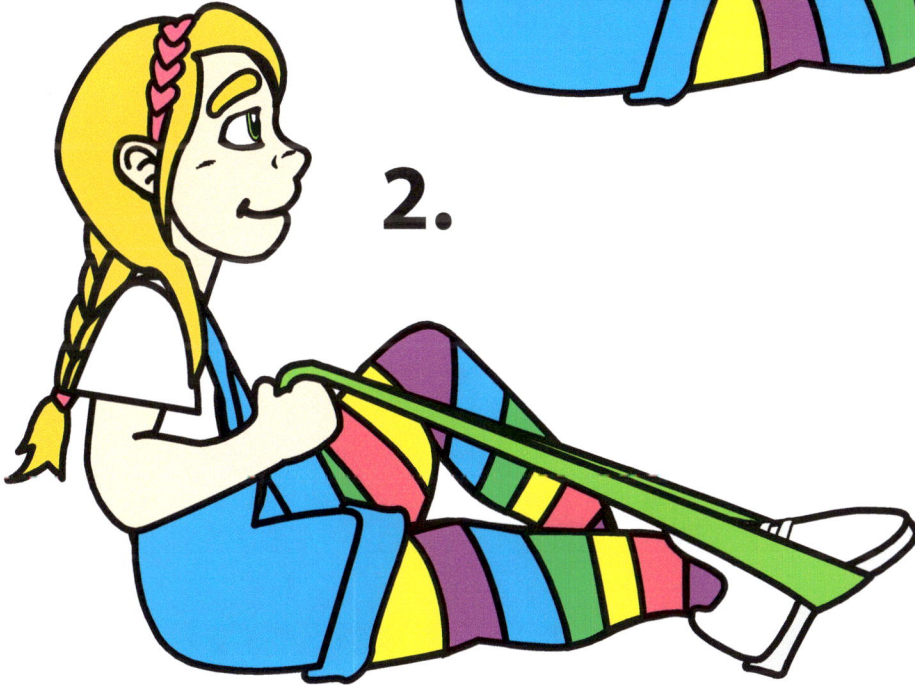

Shoulder Press

Stand up tall

Place the band under your feet

Hold the band in your hands

Raise your arms and bend your elbows

Start here and push up your arms

Touch your hands together

Slowly bring your arms back down

Can you do this 5 times?

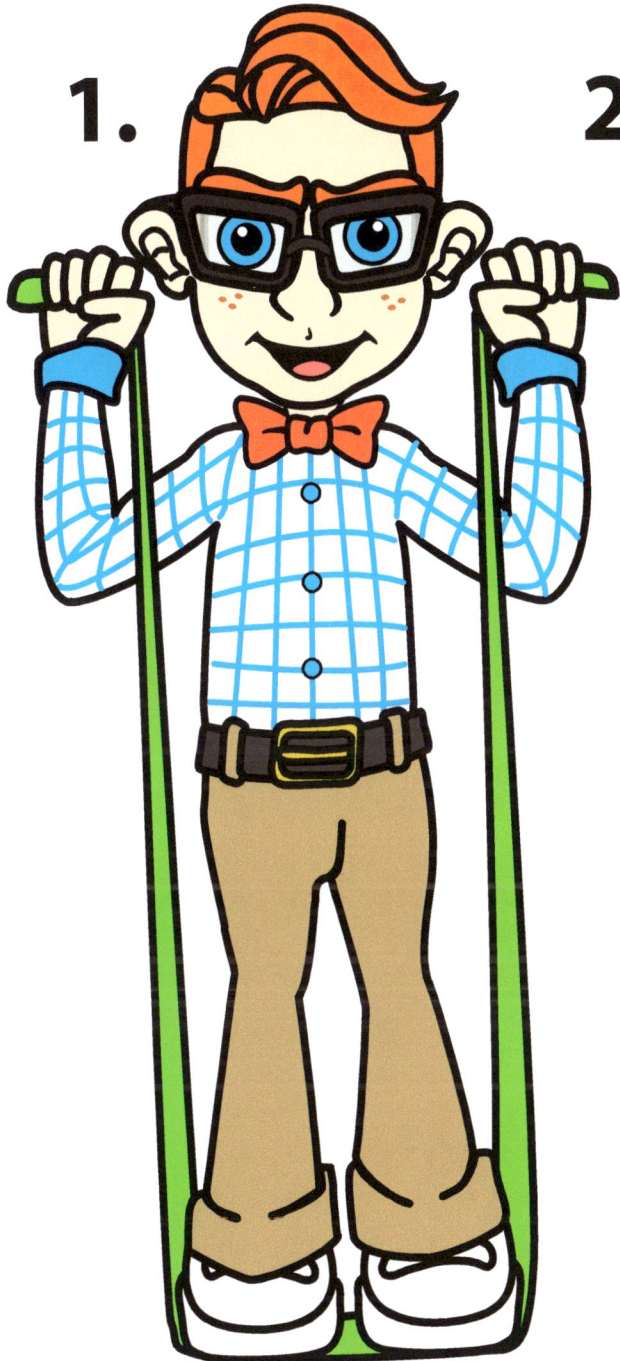

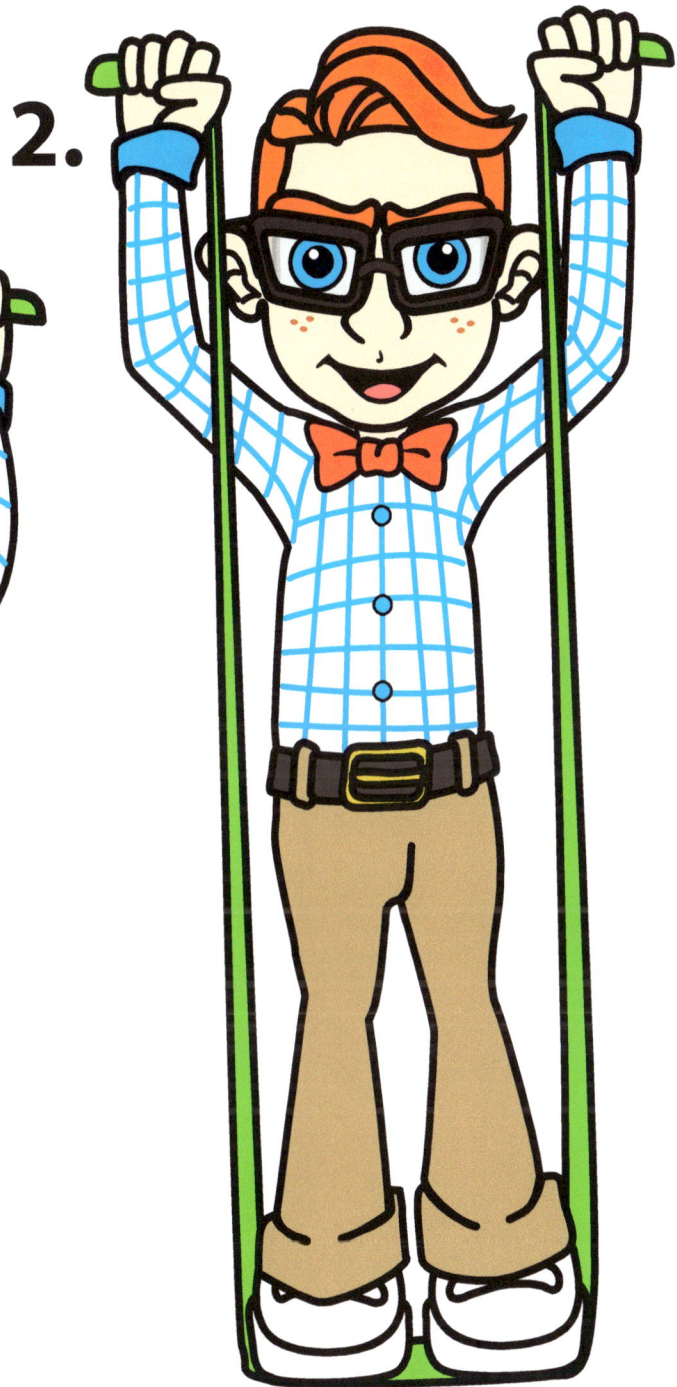

1.

2.

Seated Rows

Sit on the floor

Stretch out your legs

Place the band around your feet

Keep your legs straight

Gently pull the band back

Bend your elbows

Straighten your arms

Can you do this 5 times?

1.

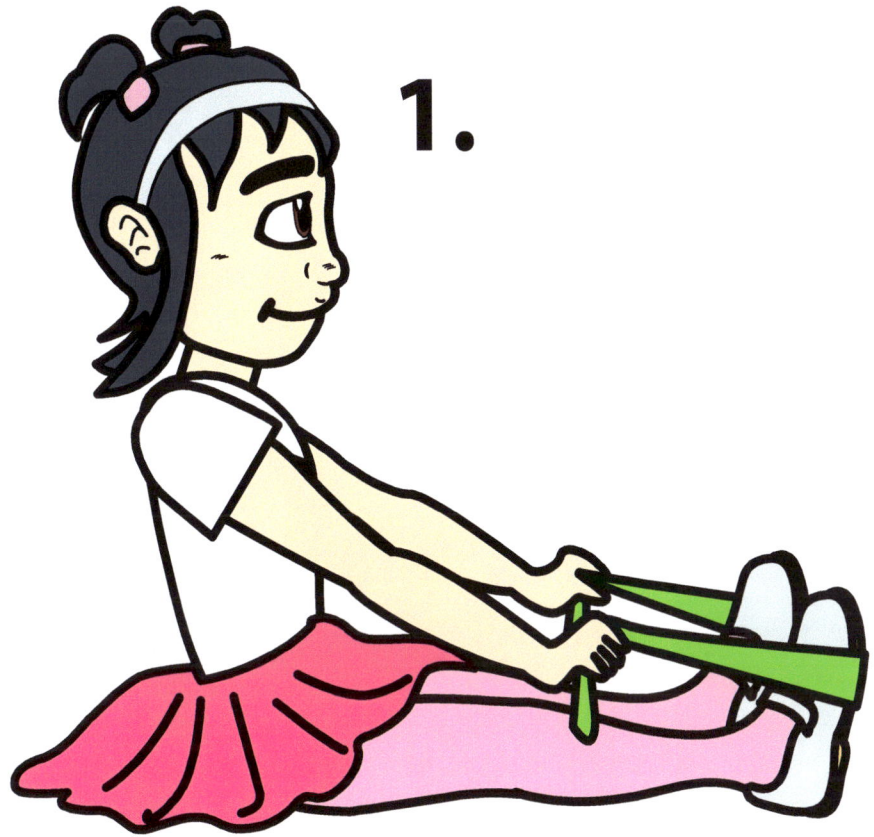

2.

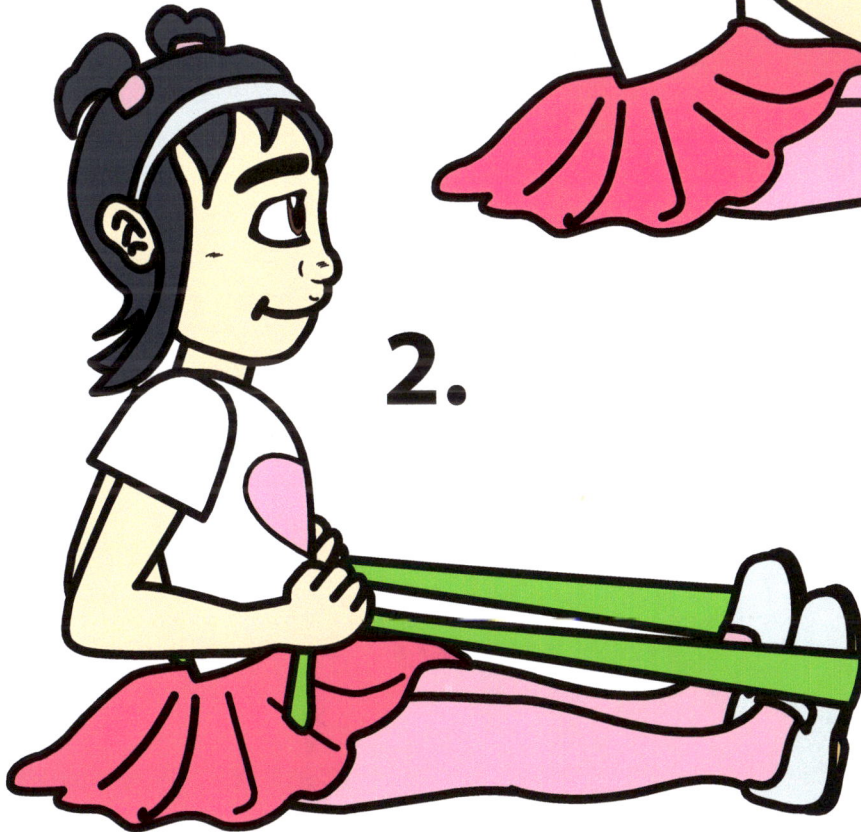

Bands 23

Bent Over Fly

Stand up straight
Bring your legs apart
Stand on the band
Bend your body over slightly
Cross over the bands with each hand
Straighten your arms out towards your feet
Pull the band with your arms out to
the sides of your body
Slowly lower your arms back down
Can you do this 5 times?

1.

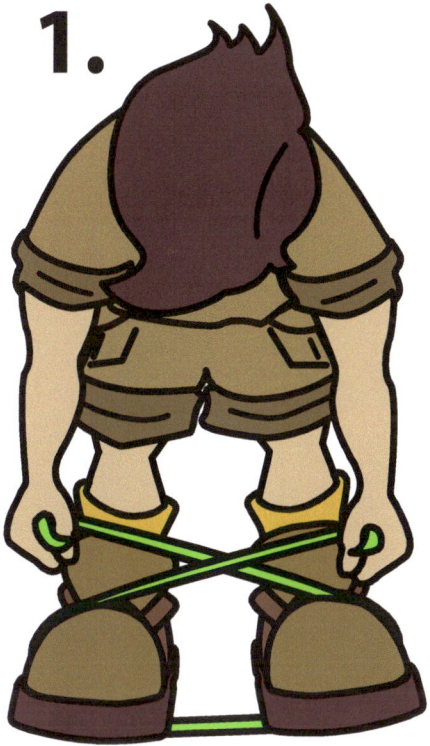

2.

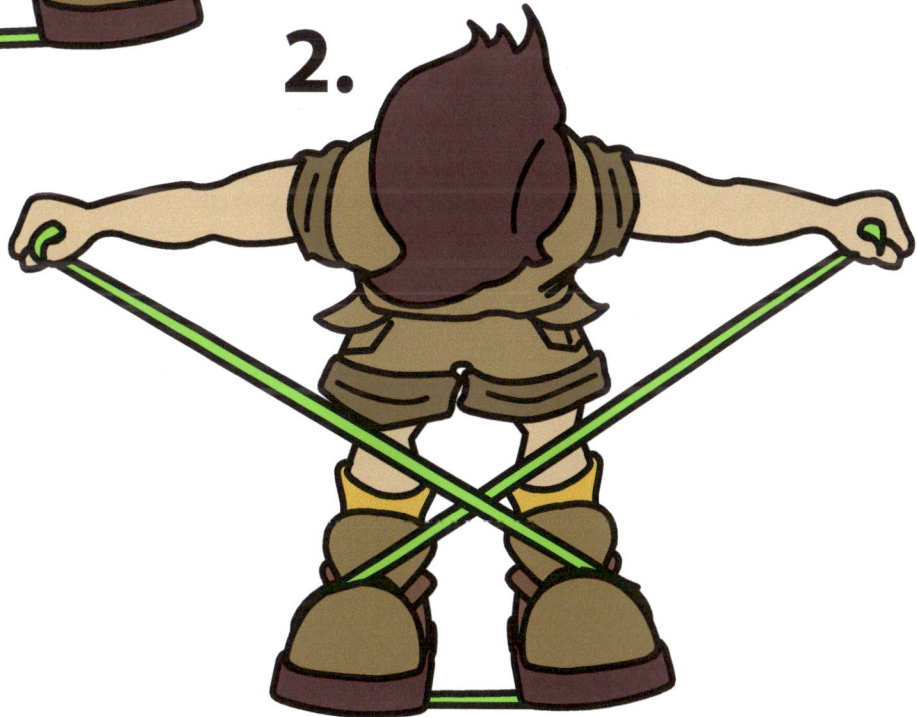

Leg Raises

Lay on your back
Place the band under your feet
Hold the band with your hands
Keep your legs straight
Keep your elbows on the floor
Slowly bring your legs up in line with your hips
Lower your legs back to the beginning
Can you do this 5 times?

1.

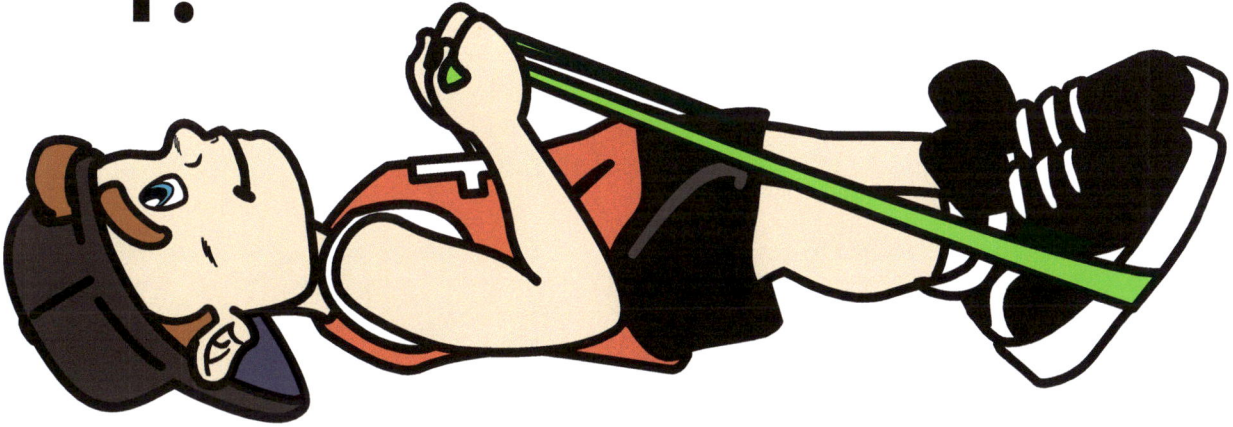

2.

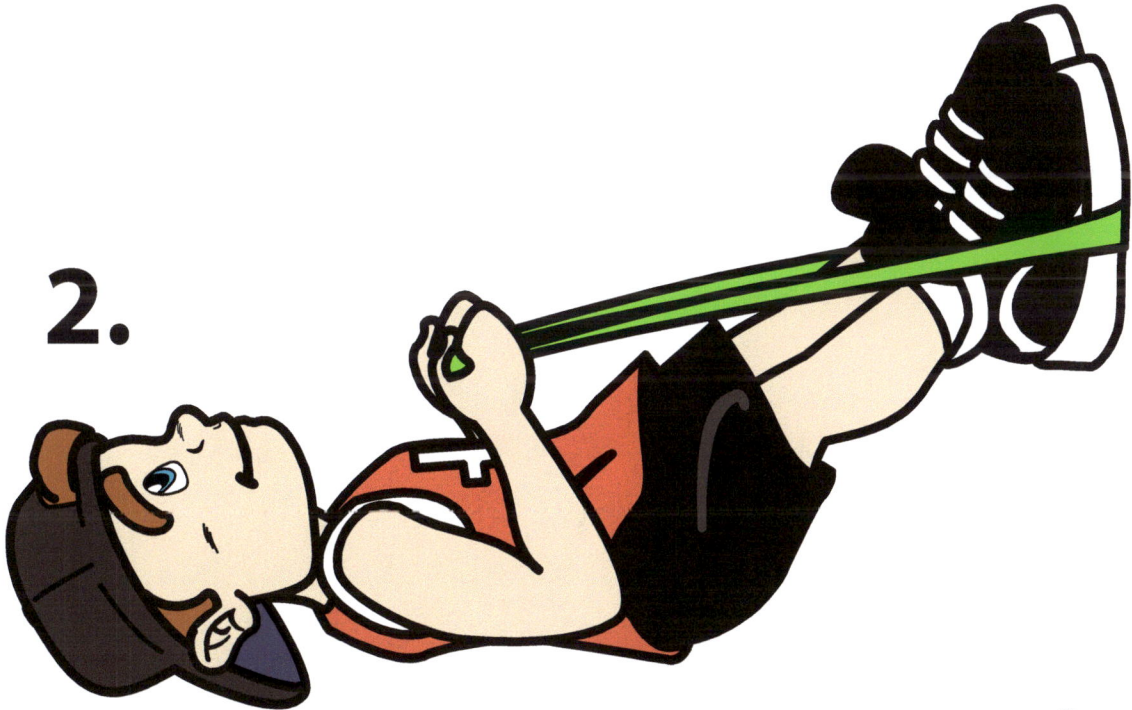

Leg Lifts

Kneel down on the floor

Place your hands down in front of you

Put the band around one foot

Keep your back straight

Slowly raise your leg up

Straighten your leg right out

Bring your leg back into the first position

Can you do this 5 times?

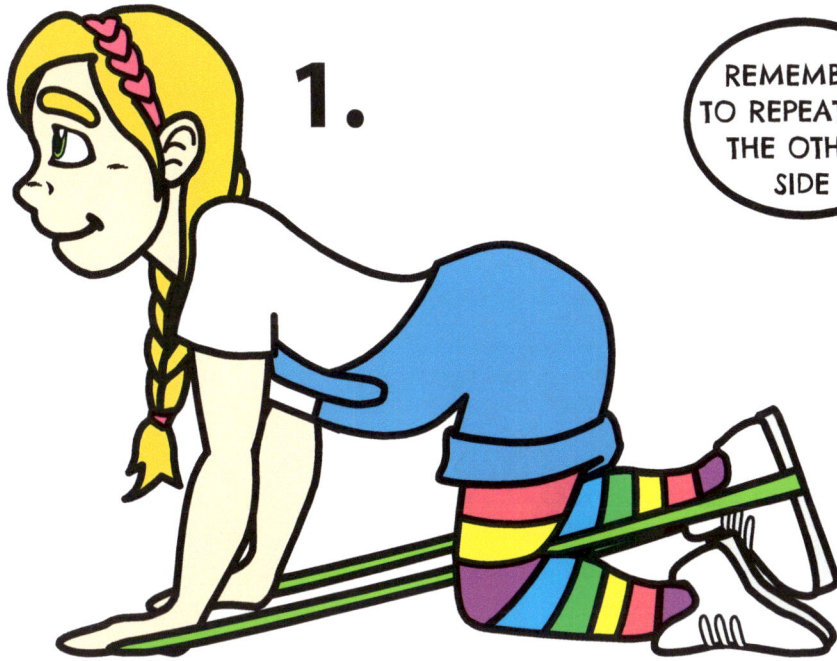

1.

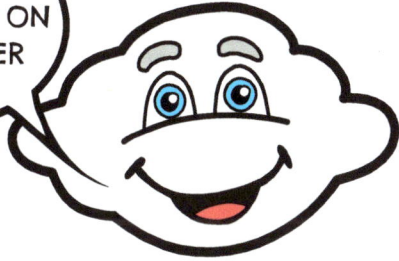

REMEMBER TO REPEAT ON THE OTHER SIDE

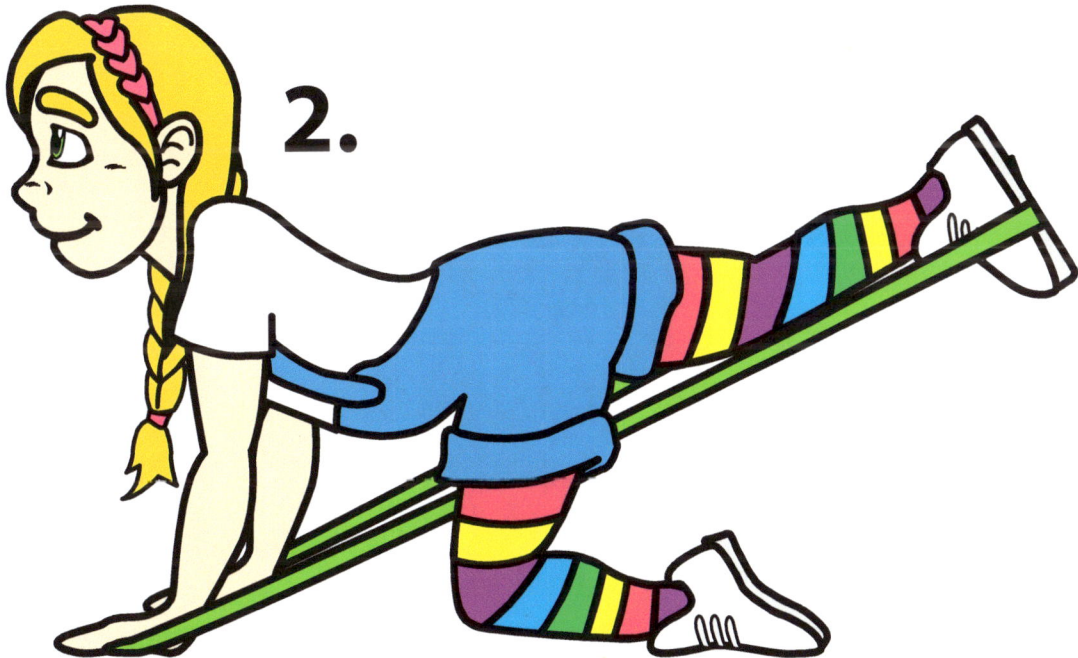

2.

Mid Back Pull

Stand up tall

Keep your legs slightly apart

Hold the band out in front of you

with both hands

Slowly stretch it out as far as you can

Keep your arms straight

Slowly bring your arms back to the first position

Can you do this 5 times?

1.

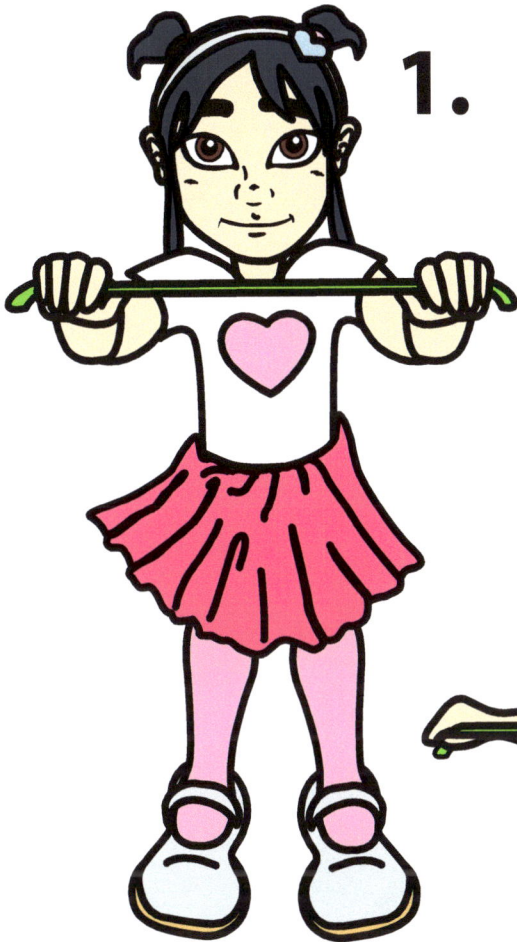

2.

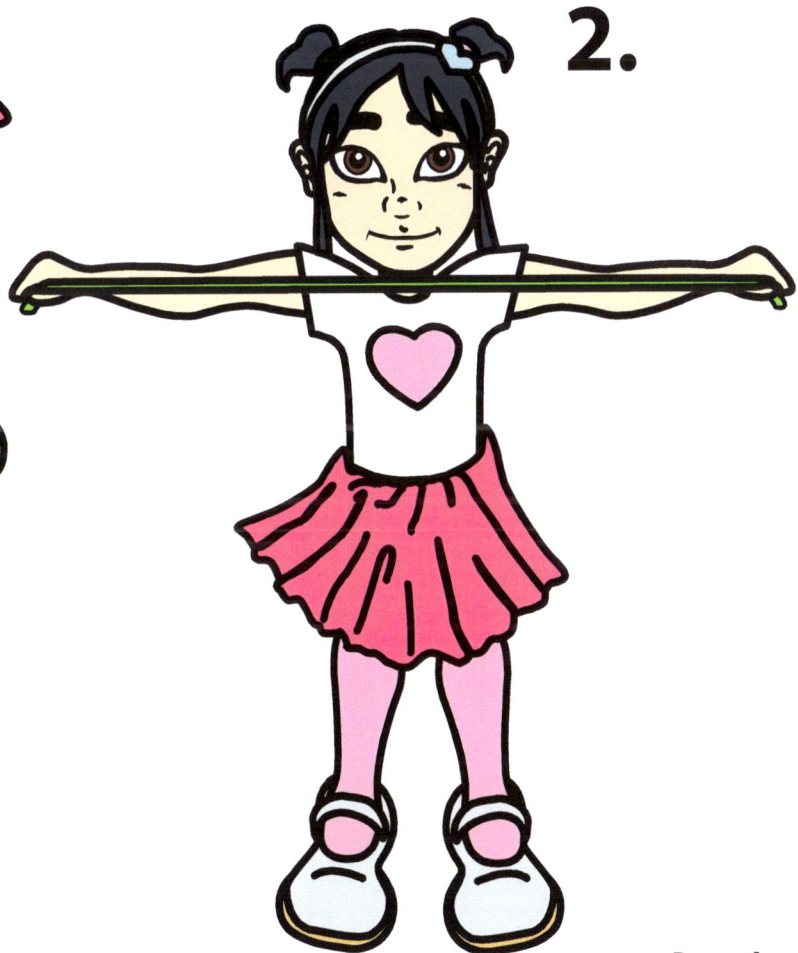

Bicep Curls

Stand up tall

Place the band under your feet

Hold the band with your hands

Keep your arms in front of your body

Slowly bend your forearms up

Keep your elbows close to your body

Lower your arms back to the start

Can you do this 5 times?

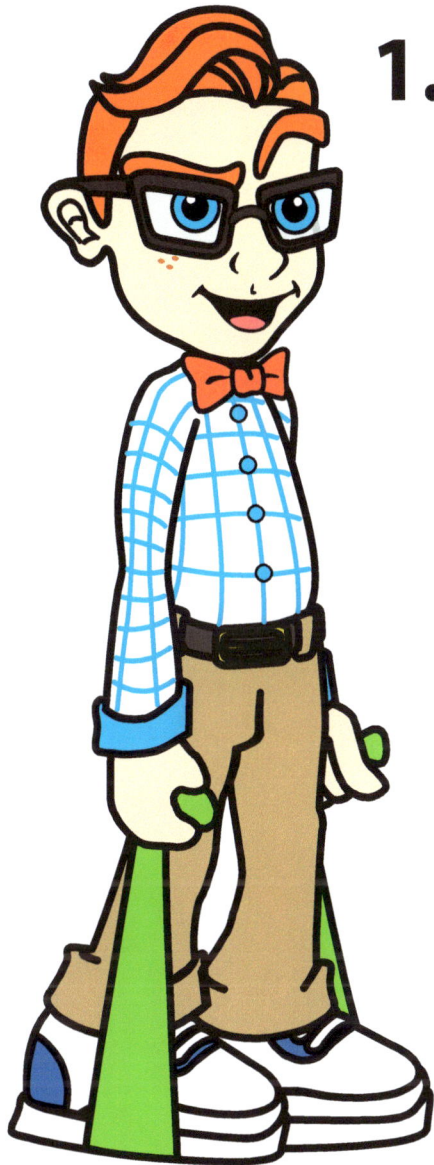

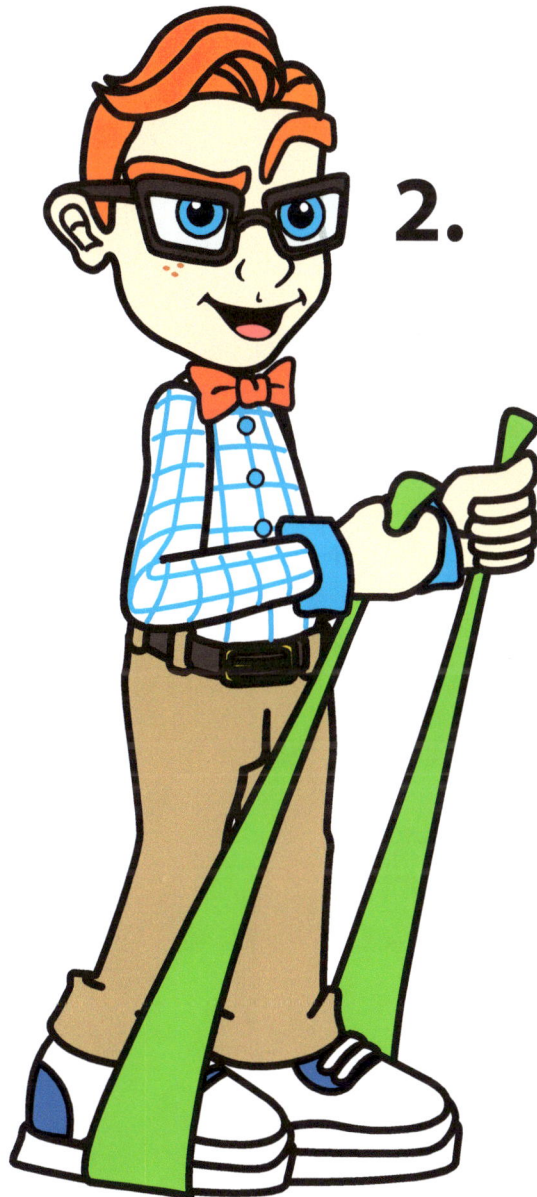

1.

2.

Squats

Stand up tall
Place your band under your feet
Hold band in your hands
Stand with feet apart
Slowly lower your body
Bend your knees
Keep your back straight
Bend only to glute is in line with knees
Slowly stand back up
Can you do this 5 times?

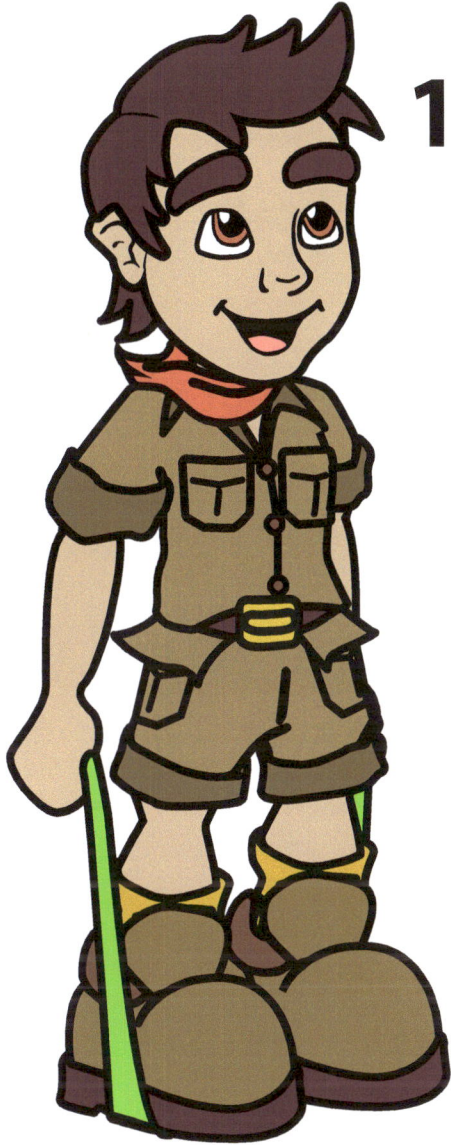

1.

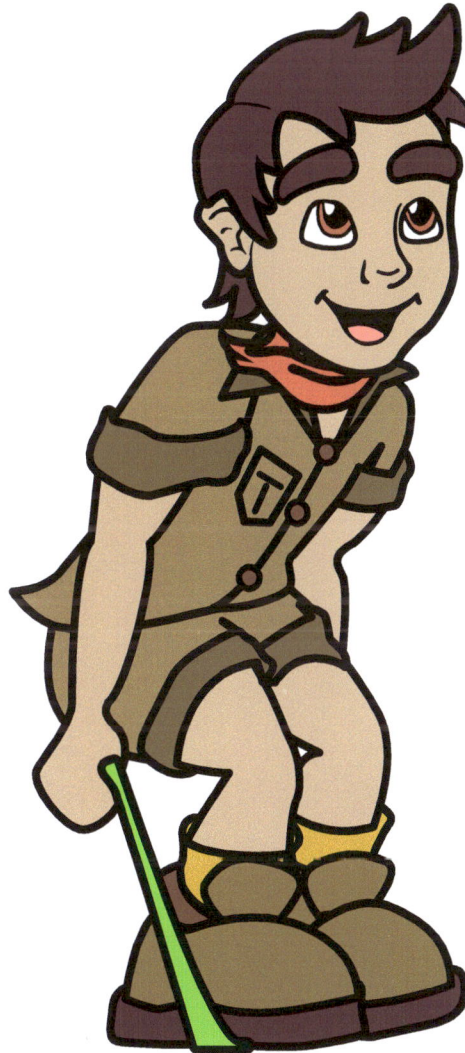

2.

Bands 35

Keep an eye out for the rest of the series

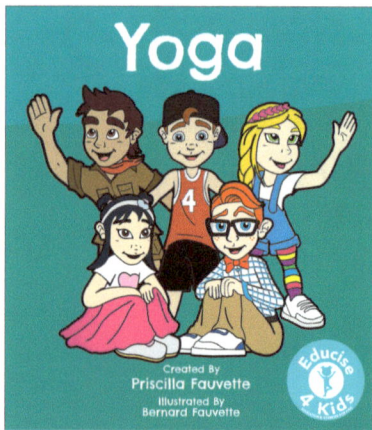

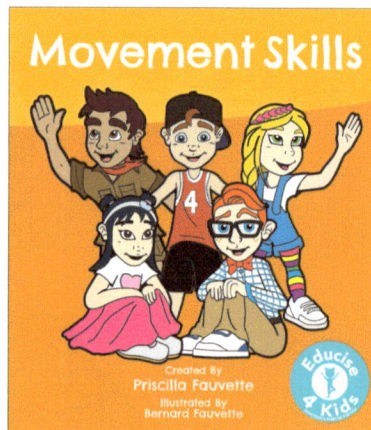

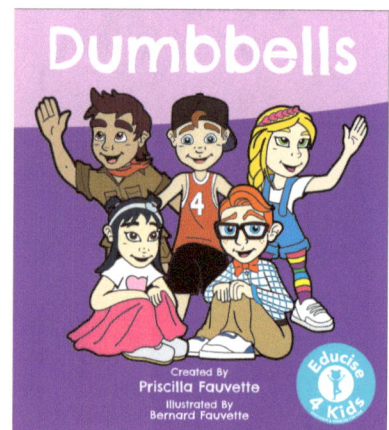

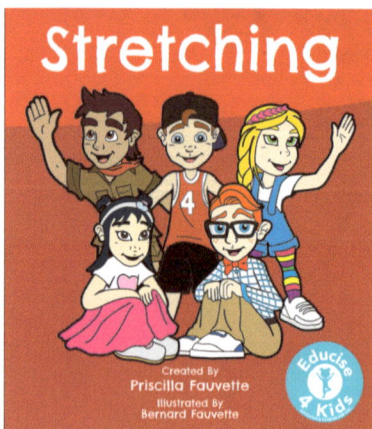

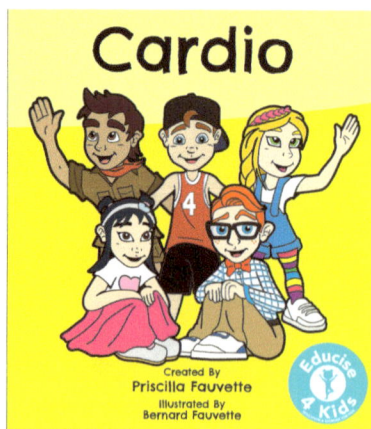

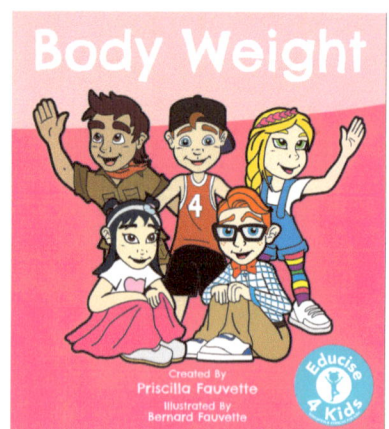

www.ingramcontent.com/pod-product-compliance
Lightning Source LLC
Chambersburg PA
CBHW061137030426
42334CB00003B/75